C000157514

TYPE _ DIABETES FOOD LIST

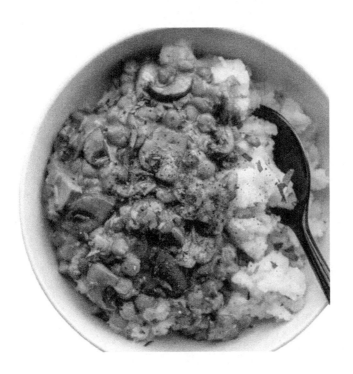

LYSANDRA QUINN

Copyright © 2023 by Lysandra Quinn

All rights reserved.

No part of this publication may be reproduced, stored in a retrieval system, or transmitted, in any form or by any means, electronic, mechanical, photocopying, recording or otherwise, without the prior written permission of the copyright holder.

This book is sold subject to the condition that it shall not, by way of trade or otherwise, be lent, re-sold, hired out or otherwise circulated without the publisher's prior consent in any form of binding or cover other than that in which it is published and without a similar condition including this condition being imposed on the subsequent purchaser.

The author has made every effort to ensure the accuracy and completeness of the Information contained in this book. However, the author and publisher assume no responsibility for errors, inaccuracies, omissions, or any inconsistency herein. Any slights of people, places or organizations are unintentional.

Contact the Author

Thank you for reading my book! I would love to hear from you, whether you have feedback, questions, or just want to share your thoughts. Your feedback means a lot to me and helps me improve as a writer.

Please don't hesitate to reach out to me through

contactmelysandraquinn@gmail.com

I look forward to connecting with my readers and appreciate your support in this literary journey. Your thoughts and comments are valuable to me.

OTHER BOOKS BY THE AUTHOR

SLOW COOKER DIABETIC RENAL COOKBOOK

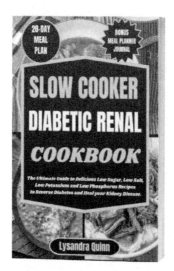

DIABETIC RENAL AIR FRYER COOKBOOK

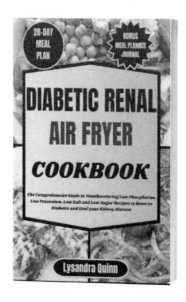

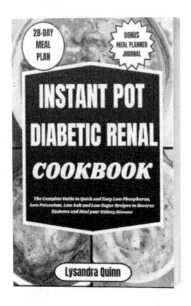

TABLE OF CONTENTS

INTRODUCTION

In the quiet corridors of life, where whispers of health concerns echo, there exists a realm shrouded in shadows—the realm of Type 2 Diabetes. It is a journey laden with uncertainty, a journey I intimately acquainted myself with as a seasoned dietician on a quest to unravel the secrets of nourishment for those grappling with this formidable adversary.

Picture this: A tapestry of lives woven together by the common thread of Type 2 Diabetes. Faces etched with frustration and disappointment, individuals who had traversed the labyrinth of food lists with hope flickering like a fragile flame. They had danced with countless diets, each promising a reprieve from the clutches of diabetes, only to find themselves ensnared in a web of unmet expectations.

For years, I delved into the vast expanse of research, a dedicated explorer seeking the golden elixir that could transform the narrative of Type 2 Diabetes. The danger it posed was not merely medical jargon; it was the silent thief stealing the joys of life, the Vigor of existence. The stakes were high, and time, unforgiving.

And then, a revelation unfolded—a mosaic of recipes that held the power to defy the status quo. These weren't just culinary concoctions; they were instruments of change, catalysts for a paradigm shift in the lives of those battling Type 2 Diabetes. The transformation was not just physical; it was a symphony of holistic well-being, a crescendo of renewed vitality.

In my role as a dietician, the journey was not merely professional—it was personal. Witnessing the metamorphosis of individuals who had grappled with the shadows of diabetes for years was nothing short of awe-inspiring. It was the birth of a mission, a resolve to distil years of research into a tangible, accessible form. The culmination of this odyssey was a food list—an offering of hope, a lifeline for those standing at the crossroads of health and despair.

This book is not a mere compilation of recipes; it is a testament to resilience, a narrative etched in the language of taste and nutrition. As you embark on this journey through the pages, envision the stories of those whose lives were touched by the alchemy of these recipes. It is a celebration of the human spirit, an ode to the triumph of discipline over disease.

But why this food list? What sets it apart from the myriad others that claim to hold the key to diabetes management? These are the questions that linger, and rightfully so. Let me pose a few more: Can you imagine a life where your relationship with food isn't defined by fear? What if the meals you savoured weren't just sustenance but a powerful ally in your battle against Type 2 Diabetes? How would it feel to bid farewell to the monotony of restrictive diets and embrace a world where flavour and health coexist harmoniously?

The advantage of this food list lies not just in its efficacy but in its simplicity—a seamless integration into the fabric of your daily life. It is a guide penned with the finesse of experience, borne out of the crucible of my 25-year-long journey as a dietician. The benefits transcend the physical realm, extending into the realms of emotional well-being and renewed vitality. It is a holistic approach, a beacon lighting the path to a life unburdened by the shadows of Type 2 Diabetes.

So, dear reader, immerse yourself in the pages that follow. Let the recipes narrate a story of rejuvenation, let the Flavors be the protagonists in a tale of triumph. This isn't just a food list; it is a lifeline, a bridge between the realms of limitation and liberation. As you Savor each recipe, remember that you are not just consuming food—you are savouring the elixir of transformation.

Welcome to a journey where taste meets triumph, where nourishment transcends the ordinary, and where the power to redefine your relationship with food rests in your hands. Together, let us embark on a culinary odyssey that whispers not just of ingredients but of possibilities—a journey where every bite is a step towards reclaiming the vitality that Type 2 Diabetes sought to steal.

CHAPTER 1

UNDERSTANDING TYPE 2

DIABETES

Type 2 diabetes is a chronic condition characterized by elevated levels of blood sugar, or glucose, in the body. Unlike type 1 diabetes, where the body does not produce insulin, individuals with type 2 diabetes either do not produce enough insulin or the body's cells become resistant to the insulin that is produced. Insulin is a hormone that helps regulate blood sugar and allows cells to use glucose for energy. When this process is impaired, it leads to an accumulation of glucose in the blood, causing various health issues.

Risk factors for type 2 diabetes include genetics, age, sedentary lifestyle, poor diet, and obesity. The prevalence of type 2 diabetes has been on the rise globally, making it crucial for individuals to understand the condition and take steps to manage it effectively.

Importance of Diet in Managing Type 2 Diabetes:

Diet plays a pivotal role in managing type 2 diabetes. A well-balanced and nutritious diet can help control blood sugar levels, maintain a healthy weight, and prevent complications associated with diabetes. When planning a diet for managing type 2 diabetes, it's essential to focus on nutrient-dense foods that provide essential vitamins and minerals without causing rapid spikes in blood sugar.

Managing carbohydrate intake is particularly crucial, as carbohydrates directly impact blood sugar levels. Choosing complex carbohydrates with a low glycemic index, such as whole grains, legumes, and vegetables, can help regulate blood sugar. Additionally, incorporating lean proteins, healthy fats, and plenty of fiber into the diet contributes to better blood sugar control and overall health.

Basic Principles of a Type 2 Diabetes Diet:

Carbohydrate Management: Monitor and control the intake of carbohydrates. Choose complex carbohydrates over simple sugars and refined grains. This includes whole grains, fruits, and vegetables.

Portion Control: Pay attention to portion sizes to avoid overeating. Controlling portion sizes helps regulate calorie intake, which is important for weight management.

Balanced Meals: Include a combination of carbohydrates, proteins, and fats in each meal. This balance helps provide sustained energy and prevents rapid spikes in blood sugar levels.

Choose Healthy Fats: Opt for sources of healthy fats, such as avocados, nuts, seeds, and olive oil. Limit saturated and trans fats, which can contribute to heart health issues.

Fiber-Rich Foods: Include plenty of fiber in the diet through whole grains, legumes, fruits, and vegetables. Fiber aids in digestion, helps control blood sugar levels, and promotes a feeling of fullness.

Regular Monitoring: Monitor blood sugar levels regularly to understand how different foods affect your body. This information can help adjust your diet and medication as needed.

Hydration: Stay well-hydrated with water and limit sugary beverages. Adequate hydration supports overall health and can aid in blood sugar management.

CHAPTER 2

BALANCING CARBOHYDRATES, PROTEINS, AND FATS

Achieving a balanced intake of carbohydrates, proteins, and fats is fundamental for maintaining overall health and supporting various bodily functions. Each macronutrient plays a unique role in the body, and finding the right balance is crucial, especially for individuals managing conditions like diabetes or those aiming for optimal health.

Carbohydrates:

Carbohydrates are the body's primary source of energy. They are found in foods like grains, fruits, vegetables, and legumes. Opt for complex carbohydrates with a lower glycemic index to provide sustained energy and help regulate blood sugar levels. Whole grains, sweet potatoes, and quinoa are examples of healthier carbohydrate choices.

Proteins:

Proteins are essential for the repair and maintenance of tissues, as well as the production of enzymes and hormones. Include lean sources of protein in your diet, such as poultry, fish, tofu, legumes, and low-fat dairy products. Balancing protein intake throughout the day can contribute to muscle health and satiety.

Fats:

Healthy fats are vital for brain function, hormone production, and the absorption of fat-soluble vitamins (A, D, E, and K). Choose sources of unsaturated fats, such as avocados, nuts, seeds, and olive oil, while limiting saturated and trans fats found in processed and fried foods. Balancing fat intake is essential for cardiovascular health.

Importance of Fiber:

Fiber is a non-digestible component of plant-based foods that provides a range of health benefits. There are two types of fiber: soluble and insoluble, both contributing to digestive health and overall well-being.

Digestive Health:

Insoluble fiber adds bulk to the stool, aiding in the movement of food through the digestive system and preventing constipation. Foods rich in insoluble fiber include whole grains, nuts, and vegetables.

Blood Sugar Regulation:

Soluble fiber helps slow the absorption of sugar, contributing to more stable blood sugar levels. This is particularly beneficial for individuals managing diabetes. Sources of soluble fiber include oats, beans, and certain fruits.

Weight Management:

High-fiber foods tend to be more filling, promoting a sense of fullness and reducing overall calorie intake. This can be advantageous for those aiming to maintain or lose weight.

Heart Health:

Fiber-rich diets are associated with a lower risk of heart disease. Soluble fiber helps lower cholesterol levels, contributing to cardiovascular health.

Portion Control:

Portion control is a key aspect of maintaining a healthy and balanced diet. It involves being mindful of the quantity of food consumed to avoid overeating and promote overall well-being.

Preventing Overconsumption:

Eating appropriate portion sizes helps prevent overconsumption of calories, which is crucial for weight management and can reduce the risk of obesity-related conditions.

Regulating Blood Sugar:

Controlling portion sizes, especially of carbohydrates, contributes to better blood sugar regulation, which is essential for individuals with diabetes or those at risk of developing the condition.

Enhancing Nutrient Intake:

Proper portion control allows for a more diverse and balanced intake of nutrients, ensuring that the body receives the necessary vitamins and minerals for optimal functioning.

Mindful Eating:

Paying attention to portion sizes encourages mindful eating, fostering a greater connection with hunger and fullness cues and promoting a healthier relationship with food.

CHAPTER 3

VEGETABLES

Spinach:

Nutritional Information (per cup):

- ✓ Calories: 7
- ✓ Carbohydrates: 1 gram
- ✓ Protein: 1 gram
- ✓ Fat: 0 grams
- ✓ Fiber: 1 gram

Broccoli:

Nutritional Information (per cup):

- ✓ Calories: 31
- ✓ Carbohydrates: 6 grams
- ✓ Protein: 3 grams
- ✓ Fat: 0 grams
- ✓ Fiber: 2.4 grams

Cauliflower:

Nutritional Information (per cup):

- ✓ Calories: 27
- ✓ Carbohydrates: 6 grams
- ✓ Protein: 2 grams
- ✓ Fat: 0 grams
- ✓ Fiber: 3 grams

Bell Peppers (Mixed Colors):

Nutritional Information (per cup):

- ✓ Calories: 46
- ✓ Carbohydrates: 9 grams
- ✓ Protein: 2 grams
- ✓ Fat: 0 grams
- ✓ Fiber: 3 grams

Zucchini:

Nutritional Information (per cup):

- ✓ Calories: 20
- ✓ Carbohydrates: 4 grams
- ✓ Protein: 1 gram
- ✓ Fat: 0 grams
- ✓ Fiber: 1 gram

Kale:

Nutritional Information (per cup):

- ✓ Calories: 33
- ✓ Carbohydrates: 6 grams
- ✓ Protein: 3 grams
- ✓ Fat: 0 grams
- ✓ Fiber: 1 gram

Brussels Sprouts:

Nutritional Information (per cup):

- ✓ Calories: 38
- ✓ Carbohydrates: 8 grams
- ✓ Protein: 3 grams
- ✓ Fat: 0 grams
- ✓ Fiber: 4 grams

Asparagus:

Nutritional Information (per cup):

- ✓ Calories: 27
- ✓ Carbohydrates: 5 grams
- ✓ Protein: 3 grams
- ✓ Fat: 0 grams
- ✓ Fiber: 3 grams

Cabbage:

Nutritional Information (per cup):

- ✓ Calories: 22
- ✓ Carbohydrates: 5 grams
- ✓ Protein: 1 gram
- ✓ Fat: 0 grams
- ✓ Fiber: 2 grams

Cucumbers:

Nutritional Information (per cup, sliced):

- ✓ Calories: 16
- ✓ Carbohydrates: 4 grams
- ✓ Protein: 1 gram
- ✓ Fat: 0 grams
- ✓ Fiber: 1 gram

CHAPTER 4

LEAN PROTEINS

Chicken Breast (Skinless, Boneless):

Nutritional Information:

- ✓ Calories: 165
- ✓ Carbohydrates: 0 grams
- ✓ Protein: 31 grams
- ✓ Fat: 3.6 grams
- ✓ Fiber: 0 grams

Turkey (Ground, 93% Lean):

Nutritional Information:

- ✓ Calories: 176
- ✓ Carbohydrates: 0 grams
- ✓ Protein: 22 grams
- ✓ Fat: 10 grams
- ✓ Fiber: 0 grams

Fish (Salmon):

Nutritional Information:

- ✓ Calories: 206
- ✓ Carbohydrates: 0 grams
- ✓ Protein: 22 grams
- ✓ Fat: 13 grams
- ✓ Fiber: 0 grams

Lean Beef (Sirloin):

Nutritional Information:

- ✓ Calories: 212
- ✓ Carbohydrates: 0 grams
- ✓ Protein: 30 grams
- ✓ Fat: 10 grams
- ✓ Fiber: 0 grams

Pork (Tenderloin):

Nutritional Information:

- ✓ Calories: 143
- ✓ Carbohydrates: 0 grams
- ✓ Protein: 25 grams
- ✓ Fat: 4 grams
- ✓ Fiber: 0 grams

Tofu:

Nutritional Information:

- ✓ Calories: 144
- ✓ Carbohydrates: 3 grams
- ✓ Protein: 16 grams
- ✓ Fat: 8 grams
- ✓ Fiber: 1 gram

Eggs:

Nutritional Information:

- ✓ Calories: 70
- ✓ Carbohydrates: 1 gram
- ✓ Protein: 6 grams
- ✓ Fat: 5 grams
- ✓ Fiber: 0 grams

Greek Yogurt (Non-fat):

Nutritional Information:

- ✓ Calories: 100
- ✓ Carbohydrates: 6 grams
- ✓ Protein: 17 grams
- ✓ Fat: 0 grams
- ✓ Fiber: 0 grams

Whole Wheat Pasta:

Nutritional Information:

- ✓ Calories: 174
- ✓ Carbohydrates: 37 grams
- ✓ Protein: 8 grams
- ✓ Fat: 1 gram
- ✓ Fiber: 6 grams

Bulgur:

Nutritional Information:

- ✓ Calories: 151
- ✓ Carbohydrates: 34 grams
- ✓ Protein: 6 grams
- ✓ Fat: 0.4 grams
- ✓ Fiber: 8 grams

Farro:

Nutritional Information:

- ✓ Calories: 337
- ✓ Carbohydrates: 71 grams
- ✓ Protein: 12 grams
- ✓ Fat: 1.7 grams
- ✓ Fiber: 11 grams

Millet:

Nutritional Information:

- ✓ Calories: 207
- ✓ Carbohydrates: 41 grams
- ✓ Protein: 6 grams
- ✓ Fat: 2 grams
- ✓ Fiber: 2 grams

Freekeh:

Nutritional Information:

- ✓ Calories: 340
- ✓ Carbohydrates: 60 grams
- ✓ Protein: 20 grams
- ✓ Fat: 2 grams
- ✓ Fiber: 12 grams

Wild Rice:

Nutritional Information:

- ✓ Calories: 166
- ✓ Carbohydrates: 35 grams
- ✓ Protein: 6.5 grams
- ✓ Fat: 0.6 grams
- ✓ Fiber: 3 grams

Dark Chocolate (70-85% Cocoa):

Nutritional Information:

- ✓ Calories: 63
- ✓ Carbohydrates: 6 grams
- ✓ Protein: 1 gram
- ✓ Fat: 4 grams
- ✓ Fiber: 2 grams

Sunflower Seeds:

Nutritional Information:

- ✓ Calories: 51
- ✓ Carbohydrates: 1.5 grams
- ✓ Protein: 1.5 grams
- ✓ Fat: 4.5 grams
- ✓ Fiber: 1 gram

CHAPTER 7

FOODS TO LIMIT OR AVOID

Sugary Beverages (e.g., Soda):

- ✓ Calories: 150
- ✓ Carbohydrates: 39 grams
- ✓ Protein: 0 grams
- ✓ Fat: 0 grams
- ✓ Fiber: 0 grams

Candy (Hard or Chewy):

- ✓ Calories: 50 (varies)
- ✓ Carbohydrates: 12 grams (varies)
- ✓ Protein: 0 grams
- ✓ Fat: 0 grams
- ✓ Fiber: 0 grams

Processed Snack Foods (Chips):

- ✓ Calories: 152
- ✓ Carbohydrates: 15 grams
- ✓ Protein: 2 grams
- ✓ Fat: 10 grams
- ✓ Fiber: 1 gram

White Bread:

- ✓ Calories: 80
- ✓ Carbohydrates: 15 grams
- ✓ Protein: 2 grams
- ✓ Fat: 1 gram
- ✓ Fiber: 1 gram

White Rice:

- ✓ Calories: 204
- ✓ Carbohydrates: 45 grams
- ✓ Protein: 4 grams
- ✓ Fat: 0 grams
- ✓ Fiber: 1 gram

Regular Pasta:

- ✓ Calories: 200
- ✓ Carbohydrates: 40 grams
- ✓ Protein: 7 grams
- ✓ Fat: 1 gram
- ✓ Fiber: 2 grams

Pastries and Baked Goods:

- ✓ Calories: Varies
- ✓ Carbohydrates: Varies
- ✓ Protein: Varies
- ✓ Fat: Varies
- ✓ Fiber: Varies

Sweetened Yogurt:

- ✓ Calories: 150
- ✓ Carbohydrates: 26 grams
- ✓ Protein: 8 grams
- ✓ Fat: 2 grams
- ✓ Fiber: 0 grams

Regular Ice Cream:

- ✓ Calories: 137
- ✓ Carbohydrates: 18 grams
- ✓ Protein: 2 grams
- ✓ Fat: 7 grams
- ✓ Fiber: 0 grams

French Fries:

- ✓ Calories: 365
- ✓ Carbohydrates: 63 grams
- ✓ Protein: 4 grams
- ✓ Fat: 14 grams
- ✓ Fiber: 6 grams

Doughnuts:

- ✓ Calories: Varies
- ✓ Carbohydrates: Varies
- ✓ Protein: Varies
- ✓ Fat: Varies
- ✓ Fiber: Varies

extension, your life? Your insights, your experiences, are the ingredients that shape the evolution of this culinary tapestry.

So, dear reader, let your feedback be the postscript to this chapter. Share your victories, your discoveries, and even your challenges. For in this exchange, we forge a community—a fellowship of those who refuse to be defined by the limitations imposed by Type 2 Diabetes.

May your culinary adventures be ever vibrant, may your journey towards health be laden with flavors that not only tantalize your taste buds but nourish your spirit. As you step into the world beyond these pages, may you carry with you not just a food list but a manifesto— a manifesto for a life where every meal is a proclamation of vitality.

Thank you for entrusting me with a slice of your journey. Until we meet again in the kitchens of well-being, savor each moment, relish each bite, and let the symphony of health play on.

BONUS:

10 TYPE 2 DIABETES RECIPES

Grilled Lemon Garlic Chicken

Cooking Time: 30 minutes

Serving: 4

Ingredients:

- ✓ 4 boneless, skinless chicken breasts
- ✓ 2 tablespoons olive oil
- ✓ 2 cloves garlic, minced.
- ✓ 1 teaspoon dried oregano
- ✓ Juice of 1 lemon
- ✓ Salt and pepper to taste

Instructions:

1. Preheat the grill to medium-high heat.
2. In a bowl, mix olive oil, garlic, oregano, lemon juice, salt, and pepper.
3. Marinate chicken breasts in the mixture for 15 minutes.
4. Grill chicken for 6-8 minutes per side until fully cooked.

Nutritional Information (per serving):

250 calories, 2g carbs, 30g protein, 14g fat, 1g fiber

Quinoa and Black Bean Salad

Cooking Time: 25 minutes

Serving: 6

Ingredients:

- ✓ 1 cup quinoa, cooked.
- ✓ 1 can black beans, drained and rinsed.
- ✓ 1 cup cherry tomatoes, halved.
- ✓ 1 cucumber, diced.
- ✓ 1/4 cup red onion finely chopped.
- ✓ 2 tablespoons olive oil
- ✓ 2 tablespoons balsamic vinegar
- ✓ Salt and pepper to taste

Instructions:

1. In a large bowl, combine quinoa, black beans, tomatoes, cucumber, and red onion.
2. In a small bowl, whisk together olive oil, balsamic vinegar, salt, and pepper.
3. Pour dressing over the salad and toss to combine.

Nutritional Information (per serving):

220 calories, 30g carbs, 8g protein, 8g fat, 6g fiber

Baked Salmon with Dill

Cooking Time: 20 minutes

Serving: 2

Ingredients:

- ✓ 2 salmon fillets
- ✓ 1 tablespoon olive oil
- ✓ 1 tablespoon fresh dill, chopped.
- ✓ 1 clove garlic, minced.
- ✓ Lemon wedges for serving.
- ✓ Salt and pepper to taste

Instructions:

1. Preheat the oven to 400°F (200°C).
2. Place salmon fillets on a baking sheet.
3. Drizzle with olive oil, sprinkle with dill, garlic, salt, and pepper.
4. Bake for 15-18 minutes until salmon is cooked through.

Nutritional Information (per serving):

300 calories, 1g carbs, 40g protein, 15g fat, 0g fiber

Cauliflower Rice Stir-Fry

Cooking Time: 15 minutes

Serving: 4

Ingredients:

- ✓ 1 head cauliflower, grated.
- ✓ 1 cup mixed vegetables (bell peppers, broccoli, carrots)
- ✓ 2 tablespoons low-sodium soy sauce
- ✓ 1 tablespoon sesame oil
- ✓ 1 clove garlic, minced.
- ✓ 2 green onions, sliced.

Instructions:

1. In a wok or large skillet, sauté garlic in sesame oil.
2. Add grated cauliflower and mixed vegetables, stir-fry for 8-10 minutes.
3. Pour soy sauce over the mixture, toss to combine.
4. Garnish with green onions before serving.

Nutritional Information (per serving):

120 calories, 15g carbs, 5g protein, 6g fat, 6g fiber

Turkey and Vegetable Skewers

Cooking Time: 20 minutes

Serving: 4

Ingredients:

- ✓ 1 pound turkey breast, cut into cubes.
- ✓ 1 zucchini, sliced.
- ✓ 1 bell pepper, cut into chunks.
- ✓ 1 red onion, quartered.
- ✓ 2 tablespoons olive oil
- ✓ 1 teaspoon dried thyme
- ✓ Salt and pepper to taste

Instructions:

1. Preheat the grill or grill pan.
2. Thread turkey, zucchini, bell pepper, and onion onto skewers.
3. In a bowl, mix olive oil, thyme, salt, and pepper.
4. Brush skewers with the mixture and grill for 8-10 minutes, turning occasionally.

Nutritional Information (per serving):

280 calories, 8g carbs, 30g protein, 15g fat, 2g fiber

Lentil and Vegetable Soup

Cooking Time: 45 minutes

Serving: 6

Ingredients:

- ✓ 1 cup dried lentils, rinsed.
- ✓ 1 onion, chopped.
- ✓ 2 carrots, diced.
- ✓ 2 celery stalks, sliced.
- ✓ 3 cloves garlic, minced.
- ✓ 1 can diced tomatoes.
- ✓ 6 cups vegetable broth
- ✓ 1 teaspoon cumin
- ✓ Salt and pepper to taste

Instructions:

1. In a large pot, sauté onion, carrots, celery, and garlic until softened.
2. Add lentils, tomatoes, vegetable broth, cumin, salt, and pepper.
3. Simmer for 30-35 minutes until lentils are tender.

Nutritional Information (per serving):

180 calories, 30g carbs, 10g protein, 2g fat, 8g fiber

Zucchini Noodles with Pesto

Cooking Time: 15 minutes

Serving: 2

Ingredients:

- ✓ 2 medium-sized zucchinis, spiralized
- ✓ 1 cup cherry tomatoes, halved.
- ✓ 1/4 cup pesto sauce
- ✓ 2 tablespoons grated Parmesan cheese
- ✓ Salt and pepper to taste

Instructions:

1. In a pan, sauté zucchini noodles until tender.
2. Toss in cherry tomatoes and pesto sauce, cook for an additional 2-3 minutes.
3. Season with salt and pepper, top with Parmesan cheese.

Nutritional Information (per serving):

220 calories, 10g carbs, 5g protein, 18g fat, 3g fiber

Asian-Inspired Broccoli and Chicken

Cooking Time: 25 minutes

Serving: 4

Ingredients:

- ✓ 1 pound chicken breast thinly sliced.
- ✓ 4 cups broccoli florets
- ✓ 2 tablespoons low-sodium soy sauce
- ✓ 1 tablespoon rice vinegar
- ✓ 1 tablespoon honey
- ✓ 1 teaspoon ginger, grated.
- ✓ Sesame seeds for garnish

Instructions:

1. In a wok or skillet, cook chicken until browned.
2. Add broccoli and stir-fry until tender-crisp.
3. In a bowl, mix soy sauce, rice vinegar, honey, and ginger.
4. Pour the sauce over the chicken and broccoli, toss until coated.
5. Garnish with sesame seeds before serving.

Nutritional Information (per serving):

280 calories, 15g carbs, 30g protein, 10g fat, 4g fiber

Roasted Vegetable Medley

Cooking Time: 30 minutes

Serving: 4

Ingredients:

- ✓ 2 cups Brussels sprouts, halved.
- ✓ 2 cups sweet potatoes, cubed.
- ✓ 1 red bell pepper, sliced.
- ✓ 1 tablespoon olive oil
- ✓ 1 teaspoon rosemary
- ✓ Salt and pepper to taste

Instructions:

1. Preheat the oven to 400°F (200°C).
2. Toss Brussels sprouts, sweet potatoes, and red bell pepper with olive oil, rosemary, salt, and pepper.
3. Roast for 25-30 minutes until vegetables are golden and tender.

Nutritional Information (per serving):

180 calories, 30g carbs, 3g protein, 7g fat, 7g fiber

Berry and Yogurt Parfait

Preparation Time: 10 minutes

Serving: 2

Ingredients:

- ✓ 1 cup Greek yogurt
- ✓ 1 cup mixed berries (strawberries, blueberries, raspberries)
- ✓ 2 tablespoons chopped nuts (almonds, walnuts)
- ✓ 1 tablespoon honey

Instructions:

1. In serving glasses, layer Greek yogurt, mixed berries, and chopped nuts.
2. Drizzle honey over the top.
3. Repeat layers and serve chilled.

Nutritional Information (per serving):

220 calories, 20g carbs, 15g protein, 10g fat, 5g fiber

Printed in Great Britain
by Amazon

44028206R00036